LOSE

THE LOVE HANDLES

Also by the author

The Runner's Book of Training Secrets

LOSE
THE LOVE
HANDLES

30 DAYS
TO AN ARROW-STRAIGHT WAIST!

Dave Kuehls

Crown Trade Paperbacks
New York

This book proposes a program of diet and physical exercise for the reader to follow. However, before starting this or any other diet and/or exercise program, you should consult your physician.

Copyright © 1996 by Dave Kuehls

Photographs by Ron Linek. Special thanks to models
Keith Laramore, Jamie Mima, and Scott Caraboolad,
and to the Baldwin-Wallace College Recreational Sports
and Services.

Published by Crown Trade Paperbacks, 201 East 50th Street,
New York, New York 10022. Member of the Crown Publishing Group.

Random House, Inc. New York, Toronto, London, Sydney, Auckland

http://www.randomhouse.com/

CROWN TRADE PAPERBACKS and colophon are trademarks of
Crown Publishers, Inc.

Printed in the United States of America

Design by Mercedes Everett

Library of Congress Cataloging-in-Publication Data is available upon request

ISBN 0-517-88795-9

10 9 8 7 6 5 4 3 2 1

First Edition

CONTENTS

LOSE
THE LOVE HANDLES

LOSE THE HANDLES, NOW!

Okay, guys. The first thing I want you to do with this book is close it.

That's right, close it. Put it down.

But first, remember these instructions. Once your hands are free, you're going to reach under your shirt and use your thumb and forefinger to pinch the flesh above your hips. Go ahead and do that. Then come back.

Okay, what'd you get? Be honest. An inch? Less? More? Did you grab a good solid chunk? Was there, in fact, so much extra flab there that you had to use your second and third finger, too?

If you pinched an inch or more, you've got yourself a set of love handles, my friend. The name is amazingly inaccurate: you don't love them, and your wife or girlfriend certainly doesn't, either. Ever hear women talk dreamily about getting their hands on your—lard?

Love handles are the number one problem area for men. Couch potatoes and dedicated athletes alike are plagued by those side pockets of fat. It's because they're so darn hard to lose. You can run, cycle, hit the stairclimber, swim, jump rope, diet, and do crunches and side bends until you're blue in the face . . . and your love handles will still be there, staring back at you in the mirror like spiteful Siamese twins.

For the most part, love handles are hard to lose because they're the first place men store fat. If you've got excess fat on your body, chances are it's made a home just above your hips. To make matters worse, love handles are generally the last fat to go when you trim down. They come easily, and they don't go down without a fight.

With this book, that's exactly what you're going to give them: a fight. *You can lose your love handles in 30 days or less.* You won't feel deprived, and you won't become a slave to the gym. This program will take some effort, but hey, some things are worth fighting for, right?

Any man who is in fairly decent shape can have an arrow-straight waist in *30 days or less* by following this simple step-by-step program.

The *Lose the Handles* program can be done at home or in the gym. Based on state-of-the-art findings and the advice of fitness and medical professionals, it is a three-pronged attack:

1• A revolutionary, highly efficient *fat-burning aerobic exercise schedule.*

2• A dynamic *weight program* **that targets the best lifts to trim your handles (it's not what you think!).**

3• A *nutritional program* **that isn't a diet—but a sensible plan where you eat to fuel your body, and trim those handles in the process.**

In each section you'll receive advice from an expert in that field. Owen Anderson, Ph.D., lent his expertise for the aerobic exercise section. Doug Lentz, Pennsylvania state director for the National Strength and Conditioning Association, provided guidance on the weight-lifting program. And we consulted Nancy Clark, author of *Nancy Clark's Sport Nutrition Guidebook,* for nutrition information. As with any exercise program, consult your physician before starting this program if you have any questions or problems.

For each day of the 30-day program, we'll tell you what exercises to do, what weights to lift, and what food to eat.

Nothing could be simpler. And it doesn't cost $89.99, like all those useless "ab" devices advertised on TV.

Use this book to lose what you gained over the holidays, or get in shape for a shirtless summer at the beach. All you

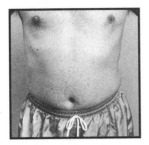

have to do is get motivated—and get to work. What do you have to lose . . . but your love handles?

Before Lose the Love Handles. *Pretty ugly, huh?*

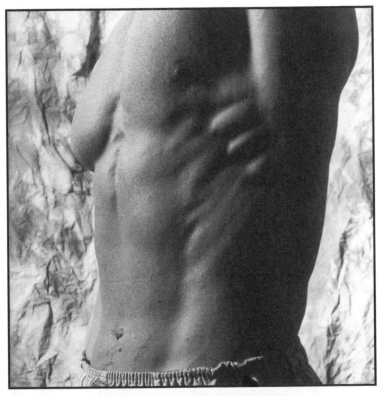

After. You can look like this in 30 days!

PART 1

THE AEROBIC EXERCISE PROGRAM

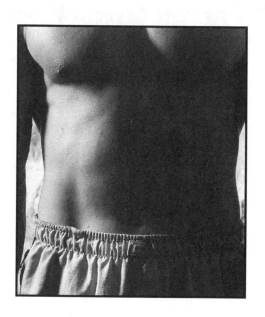

You Can't Walk Away
from Love ... Handles

"Go slow to burn fat" is the slogan that got millions of people into fitness-walking. The only problem is, it's not entirely true. Compared with fast-paced exercise, easy exercise—at 50–60 percent of maximum (more on this in sidebar on page 16) effort—burns a *higher percentage* of fat per minute, but it burns less *total fat* per minute. "You can walk off fat," says exercise physiologist Owen Anderson, Ph.D., editor of *Running Research News,* "but you'd have to do an awful lot of walking."

For example, Anderson points to a recent University of Texas study that showed that *when you exercise at 50 percent effort, fat provides 90 percent of the fuel (calories).*

Score one for slow-paced fat-burning exercise, right?

When you exercise at 75 percent effort, on the other hand, *fat provides only 60 percent of the calories.*

Score two.

But—the 75 percent effort burned more *total* fat calories per minute than the 50 percent effort: 8.4 calories compared to 6.3. In other words, vigorous exercise burned 33 percent more total fat calories per minute than slow exercise!

So, you have three choices:

1• **Spend hours a day walking off fat.**
2• **Walk only 20–40 minutes a day but accept that you'll be losing your love handles in a year, instead of 30 days.**
3• **Pick up the pace.**

I thought you'd see things the *Lose the Love Handles* way.

The revolutionary *Lose the Love Handles* aerobics component is centered around three hard workouts a week:

1• **A *Monday* "tempo" session to burn fat and get your metabolism cranking through the whole week.**

BASE FITNESS

If you're not a relatively active male (meaning you work out at least three times a week), we recommend that you take a month to put in some base aerobic conditioning before beginning this program.

A simple base-fitness program goes like this:

	M	T	W	TH	F	SAT / SUN
Week 1	10*	off	10	off	15	off
Week 2	15	off	15	off	20	off
Week 3	20	off	20	off	30	off
Week 4	25	off	25	off	40	off

During this "warm-up month" you'll build up your endurance, raise your metabolism, and gain muscular strength. By the end of the fourth week, you'll be ready to *Lose the Love Handles.*

*Minutes of easy, 50–60 percent—effort exercise—a pace where you can easily carry on a conversation. Exercise options include walking and/or jogging, stairclimbing, and cycling.

2• A *Thursday* "speed" session before and after your workout to burn fat to continue to slim down those handles.

3• A *Saturday morning* extended workout to squeeze fat out of your body, like wringing out a wet towel.

These workouts are "effort-based" so you don't have to compete with a stopwatch or partner. Go according to your own fitness level. You can use a heart monitor, or not.

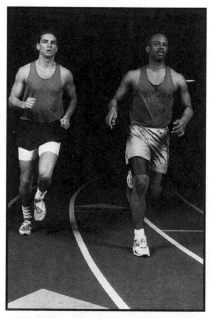

Go fast, not slow, to lose the handles.

Monday, Thursday, Saturday: The Three Fat-Burning Workouts

Monday, Tempo Time:
Burn Fat and Raise the Metabolism

You'll begin each week in the *Lose the Love Handles* program with a Monday "tempo" workout: 20–30 minutes of exercise at 85 percent effort. "Percent effort" means percentage of your maximum heart rate (MHR). To get a rough estimate of your MHR, first subtract your age from 220. Say you're 40 years old: 220 minus 40 = 180 is your maximum heart rate. Then find what 85 percent of 180 is: 153. So 153 heartbeats per minute is your "tempo" pace.

A simpler method for tempo training is this: Increase your pace to where you're beginning to breathe hard through your mouth. Slow down just a tad to get comfortable—and hold it. You've found your tempo pace.

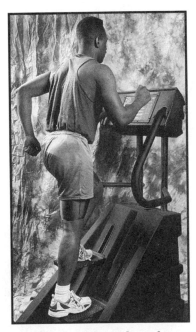

As your 20–30 minute tempo workout goes on, you might find yourself struggling to maintain pace. Don't. Remember, it's an "effort-based" workout. If you find yourself having to increase your effort to keep cycling at the same speed, slow down. *Constant effort, not speed,* is the goal of a tempo workout.

Tempo workouts burn fat and crank up your metabolism.

Wearing a heart monitor will certainly make you aware of your target heart rate. But if you don't want to use one, simply listen to your body. It'll tell you what you need to know, believe me—often in the form of tired legs or labored breathing. Your body is saying, "Slow down a little, I can't keep up the pace." Pull back some on the throttle, then keep going at your tempo pace.

SAMPLE FAT-BURNING WORKOUTS FOR ONE WEEK

MONDAY: (1) Warm up for 5 minutes with easy stepping on the stairclimber.
(2) Up the tempo to 75–85 percent effort for 20 minutes.
(3) Cool down for 5 minutes with easy stepping on the stairclimber.

THURSDAY: (1) Jog 5 minutes to warm up.
(2) Run 30 seconds at 95 percent effort. Jog for a minute. Run five times for 45 seconds at 95 percent effort with a one-minute walk in between each run.
(3) Jog 5 minutes to cool down.

FRIDAY–SATURDAY
(1) Three hours after dinner on Friday, bike 20 minutes at 60 percent effort.
(2) Before breakfast Saturday, work out on the stairclimber for 45 minutes at 70–75 percent effort.

THURSDAY, NEED FOR SPEED: BURN FAT FAST

Ever notice how lean sprinters are? They run only one lap of the track at a time—yet love handles on sprinters are nonexistent. That's because sprinters have been keeping a secret from the rest of us huffers and puffers: a secret borne out by a recent fat-burning study by Quebec's Laval University.

In the study, two groups were formed. The first group exercised continuously (it happened to be cycling, but it could just as well have been running or the stairclimber) for 30–45 minutes, five times a week, at 60 percent effort (60 percent of their MHRs).

The other group did speed work on the bike; for example, five times a week for 90 seconds at 95 percent effort. At the end of 20 weeks, researchers found that the second group—the group doing speed work—burned *almost four times* the body fat of the first.

Why? Well, researchers concluded that speed work kicked in an "after-burn" effect. That is, the body, for as long as an hour or two after exercise, burned fat as its primary energy source. In addition, they found that speed work lowers the appetite for an extended amount of time, which also leads to overall fat loss.

So to *Lose the Love Handles* on Thursday you'll be doing speed work—you guessed it—at 95 percent effort. Again, you can use a heart rate monitor, or simply exercise at a pace that's only a notch below all-out. You should be breathing very hard but maintaining a smooth cadence. Remember this phase is effort-based. If you're feeling tired by the third or fourth sprint, don't feel you need to maintain pace. Just concentrate on effort; think "quick" rather than "gut buster." At the end of your first sprint, if you find yourself, like the

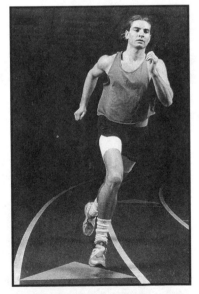

Sprint work kicks in the "after-burn" effect.

soldiers in Wilfred Owen's poem "Dulce Est Decorum Est" ("Bent double/Knock kneed/Coughing like hags"), you went way too hard.

SATURDAY, LONG AND STEADY: WRING OUT THE FAT

Saturday's fat-burning workout actually starts Friday evening. Eat an early dinner. Three hours later, do your standard recovery workout (see page 24), say, 20 minutes on the exercise bike at 60 percent effort. Drink plenty of water afterward, but go to bed without eating.

Saturday morning—*before* breakfast—exercise for 45 minutes to an hour at 75 percent effort. In other words, work out a notch or two below your Monday tempo session.

The strategy behind this dual-session is quite simple. The Friday-night workout gets your metabolism going through the night. And Saturday morning your body will be empty of carbohydrates (quick fuel for energy), so the morning workout will force your body to burn more fat than it normally would

GETTING "LAY-ED"— EFFORT LEVEL IN LAYMAN'S TERMS

Don't have a heart monitor? Here's how to gauge your level of effort during a workout. These simple guidelines explain how you feel at different levels, both physically and psychologically:

60 percent: You're on cruise control. You're enjoying the scenery or singing a song as you sweat.

75 percent: Talking is easy, but your physical efforts require some concentration.

80–85 percent: You can't talk without gasping between sentences. You need to concentrate, but you get into a groove with the pace.

95 percent: One notch below all-out effort. You're breathing hard but your action is still controlled.

and start burning fat sooner. Almost like wringing the fat from your body.

Option Plays: What Exercises to Choose and Why

The Monday, Thursday, and Saturday workout exercises in the *Lose the Love Handles* program were chosen with two criteria in mind: ease of use and calorie-burning ability.

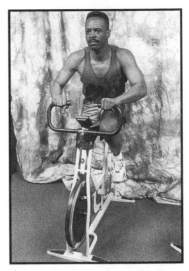

A long, steady session on the bike will force your body to rely on fat for fuel.

Obviously, if you live in Miami you're not going to get much out of a program that emphasizes cross-country skiing and speed skating (two exercises that burn lots of calories). Similarly, not everyone can play 40 straight minutes of basketball three times a week—because they can't find a court, don't know nine other guys, or couldn't hit a layup if their lives depended on it. Almost any man can accomplish the exercises in this program—running, cycling, stairclimber—with a minimum of talent, equipment (shoes, bike, membership to a gym), and hassle (you don't have to wait for a specific exercise class, lane, or group of people).

Running, cycling, and stairclimbing are three of the most effective calorie burners (see chart, page 26).

Running

Running is the simplest, but in many ways the hardest exercise for some people. You need *good* running shoes—not

WARMING UP TO IT—AND COOLING OFF

Warm-ups and cool-downs are simple, but they are vitally important to the *Lose the Love Handles* program.

Warm-ups: Five minutes of jogging, easy cycling, or walking gets the cardiovascular system going and the muscles loosened up. In short, it prepares your whole body for the stress of the tempo run or interval session.

Without warming up, stress hits an unprepared body—and that can cause injury. Think of your body as a cold car on a January morning. You wouldn't turn the key and floor the thing—you'd give it a chance to warm up.

Cool-downs: Five minutes of easy jogging or cycling or walking relaxes the body, lets the cardiovascular system wind down, and lets tired muscles ease back to a resting state. It also flushes from your muscles waste products that have accumulated during the workout, easing next-day stiffness or soreness. To use the car analogy again: you wouldn't cut the engine doing 85 on the highway, would you?

A good warm-up and a cool-down of 5 minutes of easy walking is key.

basketball or tennis shoes or some cheapo jogging model that costs $19.99. Good running shoes are made specifically for that purpose, are manufactured by well-known shoe companies, and will cost you $65–$70, minimum. The investment is worth it, too, if you want to avoid knee pain or ankle soreness or foot problems that can come from wearing the wrong shoes or poorly constructed shoes.

Loose-fitting shorts and a shirt or sweatshirt (for outside running) are the only other pieces of equipment you'll need. Some keys to running:

1 • Hold your arms waist-to rib-cage–level. Any higher and you'll tighten your shoulders and eventually your whole body.
2 • Don't ball your fists. Keep your hands loose.
3 • Stride naturally. Every runner has a unique stride.
4 • Start out slowly. Sprinting as soon as you get to the track will bring on tired muscles fast, and can cause injury.

CYCLING

Biking is easy, effective, and less stressful on your joints than running. Bike shorts with padding on the butt are recommended to prevent "saddle sores."

Some keys to cycling:

1 • Adjust your seat so that your legs are straight at the bottom of each pedal stroke.

TIME, TIME
TICKING . . .

In the *Lose the Love Handles* program, we advise evening and after-work sessions: a time when most of you have some time. Evening workouts also give you something to look forward to at the end of the day. But if you're pressed for time, most of these workouts are short enough to be done during your lunch hour or before work. The key is *consistency*. So, rather than skip a key session because you've got tickets to the game after work or an early dinner date, try to squeeze it in during the day.

2• **Lean forward and grip the handlebars lightly but securely.**

3• **Start slowly.**

Stairclimber

Good luck getting on a stairclimber during peak hours at the gym. A favorite machine since it first hit the scene in the late '80s, the stairclimber is less damaging to joints than running, but gives you a great workout anyway. Wear your running shoes, shorts, and shirt.

Some keys to stairclimbing:

1• **Keep your body as upright as possible.**

2• **Grip the side rails lightly for balance, not support.**

3• **Or swing your arms in a running motion if you can maintain balance.**

4• **Start slowly.**

Tuesday, Wednesday, Friday, Sunday: Rest and Recovery

All work and no rest and recovery makes Jack a sore and tired boy—someone who won't be able to make it to even the second week of the *Lose the Love Handles* program. That's why each week is set up so that you have *more* easy days (4) than hard days (3). Our ultimate goal is not only to lose your love handles, but to get you in such good shape that you can keep them off, permanently.

And you can only do that if you know when to push it and know when to back off. (A workout secret is that your body gets stronger on recovery or rest days—not on your hard workout days.) Consider every Tuesday, Wednesday, and Friday as a recovery workout. Choose something short

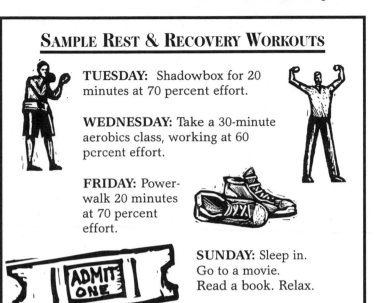

SAMPLE REST & RECOVERY WORKOUTS

TUESDAY: Shadowbox for 20 minutes at 70 percent effort.

WEDNESDAY: Take a 30-minute aerobics class, working at 60 percent effort.

FRIDAY: Power-walk 20 minutes at 70 percent effort.

SUNDAY: Sleep in. Go to a movie. Read a book. Relax.

(20–30 minutes total) and easy (60–70 percent of your MHR): something that will keep your metabolism cranking (and burning fat), but will also leave you refreshed and ready for hard workouts on Monday, Thursday, and Saturday.

Make sure you observe Sunday as a day completely off. Yes, a day off. Two-time Olympic marathoner Ed Eyestone has taken every Sunday off for fifteen years. He says it has made him stronger, plus kept his body at a high fitness level without breaking down.

Use Tuesdays, Wednesdays, and Fridays as days to experiment; try something different or funky in the way of aerobic exercise. The *Lose the Love Handles* program includes exercise options for these days such as boxing, aerobics (got your eye on the brunette in the front of the exercise studio?), skipping rope, rowing, even power walking. Make sure you spice up your weekly schedule so it won't seem so much like a routine, but like something you want to do.

BURN, BABY, BURN: CALORIE BURNERS

Activity & Calories Burned in 30 Min. (160 lb. man)

Aerobics	312	(1¼ slice pizza)	Skipping rope	288	(1¹⁄₁₀ slice pizza)	
Baseball/ Softball	178	(⁷⁄₁₀ slice pizza)	Rowing	432	(1⁷⁄₁₀ slice pizza)	
Basketball	303	(1¼ slice pizza)	Running			
Boxing	380	(1½ slice pizza)	Easy	330	(1³⁄₁₀ slice pizza)	
Calisthenics	158	(⅗ slice pizza)	Vigorous	547	(2⅕ slice pizza)	
Cycling			Stairclimber			
Easy	158	(⅗ slice pizza)	Easy	300	(1⅕ slice pizza)	
Vigorous	340	(1½ slice pizza)	Vigorous	432	(1⁷⁄₁₀ slice pizza)	
Handball	307	(1¼ slice pizza)	Swimming	336	(1³⁄₁₆ slice pizza)	
Hiking	192	(⅘ slice pizza)	Tennis	307	(1⅕ slice pizza)	
Judo/ Karate	412	(1⅗ slice pizza)	Volleyball	144	(⅗ slice pizza)	
Racquetball	312	(1⅕ slice pizza)	Walking	216	(⅘ slice pizza)	

Variety: The Spice to Lose Those Love Handles

No one said the *Losing the Love Handles* program was going to be easy or entertaining. It's not something you do 8 minutes a day while watching TV. Losing your love handles is going to take work, and any program that promises otherwise should be regarded with a highly skeptical eye.

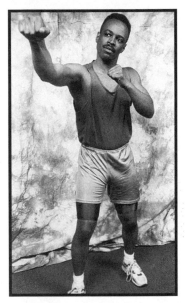

Knock out love handles with shadowboxing.

That said, there are ways to make these exercises less taxing. For example, steady runs (like your Monday tempo session) can be done on a park trail instead of a track (going around in circles can get monotonous) or treadmill (going nowhere at a steady pace can be boring). Save the track or treadmill for your Thursday speed workout. The businesslike atmosphere will get you seriously ready to burn some fat.

Ditto for cycling: Tempo rides can be done on country roads or park trails; use the stationary bike for intervals.

The stairclimber? Your options are more limited. But at your gym try to choose a stairclimber that isn't facing a blank wall. And pick a time to work out when there are a few people around to talk to.

As for your recovery days, keep things interesting. Don't fall into a rut. We've given you a number of suggestions (choose from the chart on page 26) to keep things interesting.

LOSE THE Love HANDLES EXERCISE PROGRAM

Day 1 Monday: Tempo
Warm up with 5 minutes of easy cycling.
Cycle for 20 minutes at 85 percent effort.
Easy cycling for 5 minutes to cool down.

Day 2 Tuesday: Recovery
20 minutes of easy effort exercise (choose
from: boxing, skipping rope, aerobics,
rowing machine, power walking).

Day 3 Wednesday: Recovery
25 minutes of easy effort
exercise (choose from: boxing,
skipping rope, aerobics, rowing
machine, power walking).

Day 4 Thursday: Speed
Warm up with 10 minutes of
easy jogging. Run 4 times for
60 seconds at 90–95 percent
effort with a 2-minute walk/jog
in between each. Easy jogging for
10 minutes to cool down.

**Day 5 Friday: Recovery
(preparation for Saturday)**
After dinner: 30 minutes
easy effort exercise (choose
from: boxing, skipping rope,
aerobics, rowing machine,
power walking).

The need for speed.

Day 6 Saturday: Long and Steady
Before breakfast cycle 50 minutes at 75
percent effort.

Day 7 Sunday: Rest
Go to a movie, take a nap, pet the dog.

Day 8 Monday: Tempo
Warm up with 5 minutes of easy
stepping on the stairclimber.
Step for 23 minutes at 85 percent effort.
Cool down with 5 minutes of
easy stepping.

Day 9 Tuesday: Recovery
20 minutes of easy effort exercise
(choose from: boxing, skipping rope,
aerobics, rowing machine, power
walking).

Day 10 Wednesday: Recovery
25 minutes of easy effort exercise
(choose from: boxing, skipping,
rope, aerobics, rowing machine,
power walking).

Day 11 Thursday: Speed
Easy jogging 10 minutes to warm up.
Run 5 times for 60 seconds at 90–95
percent effort with a 2-minute walk/jog
between each.
Easy jogging for 10 minutes to cool down.

**Day 12 Friday: Recovery
(preparation for Saturday)**
After dinner: 20 minutes of easy
effort exercise (choose from: boxing,
skipping rope, aerobics, rowing machine,
power walking).

Day 13 Saturday: Long and Steady
Before breakfast, cycle 60 minutes at
75 percent effort.

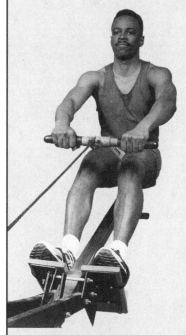

Day 14 Sunday: Rest
Watch a ball game, meet
for brunch, pet the cat.

Day 15 Monday: Tempo
Easy jogging for 5 minutes
to warm up.
Run 27 minutes at 85
percent effort.
Easy jogging for 5 minutes
to cool down.

**Day 16 Tuesday:
Recovery**
25 minutes of easy
effort exercise (choose
from: boxing, skipping
rope, aerobics, rowing
machine, power
walking).

Row off the handles.

Day 17 Wednesday: Recovery
20 minutes of easy effort exercise (choose from: boxing, skipping rope, aerobics, rowing machine, power walking).

Day 18 Thursday: Speed
Easy jogging for 10 minutes to warm up. Run 6 times for 60 seconds at 90–95 percent effort with a 2-minute walk/jog in between each.
Easy jogging for 10 minutes to cool down.

Day 19 Friday: Recovery
(preparation for Saturday)
After dinner: 20 minutes of easy effort exercise (choose from: boxing, skipping rope, aerobics, rowing machine, power walking).

Day 20 Saturday: Long and Steady
Before breakfast: stairclimber for 60 minutes at 75 percent effort.

Day 21 Sunday: Rest
Have a picnic, hang out at a coffee shop, read the *whole* newspaper.

Day 22 Monday: Tempo
Easy cycling for 5 minutes to warm up. Cycle 30 minutes at 85 percent effort. Easy cycling for 5 minutes to cool down.

Day 23 Tuesday: Recovery

20 minutes of easy effort exercise (choose from: boxing, skipping rope, aerobics, rowing machine, power walking).

Day 24 Wednesday: Recovery

20 minutes of easy effort exercise (choose from: boxing, skipping rope, aerobics, rowing machine, power walking).

Day 25 Thursday: Speed

Easy jogging for 10 minutes to warm up. Run 7 times for 60 seconds at 90–95 percent effort with a 2-minute walk/jog in between each. Easy jogging for 10 minutes to cool down.

Day 26 Friday: Recovery (preparation for Saturday)

After dinner: 20 minutes of easy effort exercise (choose from:

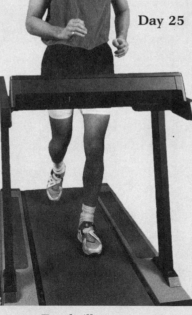

Treadmill your way to an arrow-straight waist.

boxing, skipping rope, aerobics, rowing machine, power walking).

Day 27 Saturday: Long and Steady
Before breakfast: cycle 60 minutes at 75 percent effort.

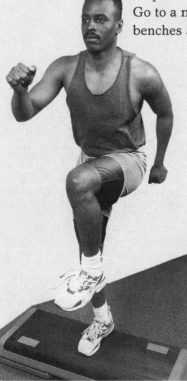

Day 28 Sunday: Rest
Go to a museum—but sit on benches a lot; buy a new CD; get a massage.

Day 29 Monday: Tempo
Easy 5 minutes on the stairclimber to warm up.
30 minutes on the stair-climber at 85 percent effort.
Easy 5 minutes on the stairclimber to cool down.

Day 30 Tuesday: Recovery
20 minutes of easy effort exercise (choose from: boxing, skipping rope, aerobics, rowing machine, power walking).

Step up to aerobics.

PART 2

THE WEIGHT TRAINING PROGRAM

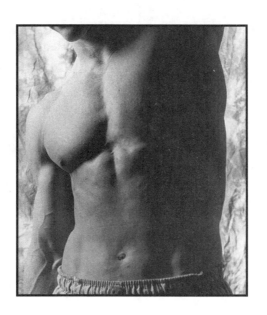

DOUBLE-TROUBLE FOR LOVE HANDLES

Walk into any health club or gym, and you'll see guys with noticeable love handles lining up at the ab machine. Or they're down on the floor, clutching weights to their chests like life preservers doing sit-up after sit-up after sit-up. The next day they're at it again—and again, and again. Some guys have been doing this for years. And they still haven't taken one inch off their love handles.

This next sentence may permanently change the way you think about exercise. The truth is—

Spot reduction doesn't work.

I'll repeat: Spot reduction doesn't work.

Doing sets on the ab machine, sit-ups, side bends, and crunches with weight plates in order to lose your love handles is like massaging the top of your head to get taller. "Fat loss is a whole-body process," says Doug Lentz, Pennsylvania state director for the National Strength and Conditioning Association. "The minimal fat you burn doing side bends doesn't have to come from your side, even though that's the area you're working out. Your body is going to pull fat from wherever it wants to, not wherever *you* want it to."

At best, abdominal work will firm and tone the abdominals and the obliques muscles on the sides of your stomach. "But if you've got a lot of fat hanging there, guess what you see?" says Lentz.

Right. Fat. Sitting right on top of your abs of steel.

Now the good news. Weight training can help you lose your love handles. But it has to be the *right kind of weight training,* the kind that both burns maximum fat during your workout and adds muscle to your body that cranks up your resting metabolism so you will burn more fat all the time, even at rest. For every new pound of muscle you gain, you burn approximately 75 more calories each day.

SLOW
AND STEADY
WINS THE RACE:
LIFT TO MAXIMIZE
FAT LOSS
AND MUSCLE GAIN

Grunting and jerking weights around quickly might get you stared at—but won't burn a whole lot of fat or build much muscle. Experts on weight lifting agree that slow and steady wins the race when it comes to losing fat and building muscle.

A good rule of thumb is to **count to two when you bring a weight up and four when you put it down.** Lift in a controlled fashion: Don't swing the weights or move without control.

Slow, controlled lifting puts the focus on one specific muscle or muscle group, which causes that muscle to work harder—and, ultimately, to grow. An analogy is painting a wall with slow, steady strokes that cover the wall efficiently, instead of short, quick strokes, which spatter paint around.

BIG MUSCLES, BIG FAT LOSS

The *Lose the Love Handles* weight program focuses on the larger muscle groups, including the butt and thighs, chest area, and back. The reasoning? These muscles burn more calories—and fat— during and after a workout than do the smaller muscle groups.

The *Lose the Love Handles* weight program targets two intense weights sessions each week (coordinated with the aerobics program to follow a hard workout on the exercise bike, stairclimber, or treadmill). Each weights session will focus on the large muscle groups, maximizing fat loss and muscle gain. There will be some spot work on the love handles area, but it will be a *part* of the *total* program: toning the zone so that when the fat melts off your hips, your hips are worth showing off.

In a related issue, the last body part you want to concentrate on when you're trying to trim your love handles is your arms. That's right. Think of all those Joey Buttafuoco look-alikes with rock-solid biceps and basketball-sized bellies and you begin to get the picture. "Guys don't want to hear this," Doug Lentz says, "but big arms don't burn much fat." So while we do include biceps and triceps in this program, they are only a small part of it.

The *Lose the Love Handles* weight program is a circuit workout; that is, you'll be going from one lift to another as quickly as possible. "Circuits work really well to burn fat and give you a cardiovascular workout at the same time," Lentz says. "Plus, they're very time efficient."

Circuits can be done in your home or at the gym or health

A POUND OF FLESH

Muscle growth is like preventative medicine in the battle against love handles. For each pound of muscle you add, your resting metabolism rises by roughly 75 calories per day. In 30 days, then, your body burns an extra 2,450 calories just sitting around. Sounds like a tabloid headline, but it's true: LOSE 3/4 LB. OF FAT IN ONE MONTH WHILE YOU WATCH TV OR READ A BOOK!

club, on machines or with free weights. The idea is to go directly from one lift to the other, doing 10 to 15 reps on each until you have completed all lifts in the circuit. Then repeat the whole circuit one or two more times. On the following pages you will see one circuit option if you're working with free weights, and the equivalent circuit performed on machines at the gym.

THE LOSE THE LOVE HANDLES CIRCUIT: FREE WEIGHT OPTION

Do one set of 10–15 repetitions of each exercise. Then repeat entire circuit 1–2 more times.

To find the weight that's right for you on each lift, first experiment with very light weights, working your way up to a weight that you can lift at least 10 times—but not more than 15 times. That's a good starting weight. Then, when you can easily lift that weight 15 times, add a few pounds.

1. Squats

Stand upright with a barbell behind your head and across your shoulders. Bend at the hips and knees, keeping your back straight as you lower yourself into a squatting position. Then come back up. Remember, as you do this exercise (and all those that follow), think of keeping your stomach muscles pulled in nice and tight (to avoid straining your back) and never lock your knees.

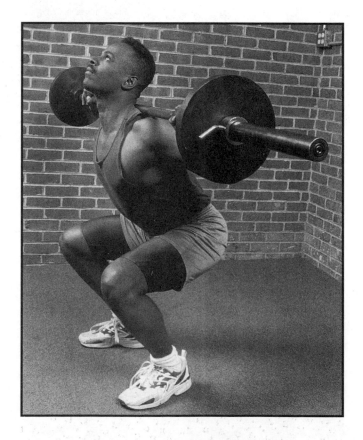

2. Dead Lift

With the barbell on the floor in front of you, bend slightly at the knees and grip the bar with hands a little more than shoulders-width apart. Stand up smoothly. Pause. Lower barbell smoothly to the floor.

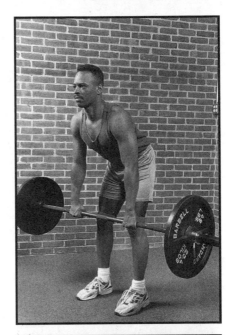

3. Calf Raise

With a barbell resting across your shoulders behind your head, stand straight, feet shoulders-width apart, and raise yourself up on your toes. Pause. Then lower weight.

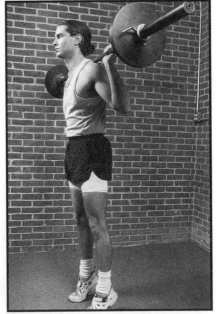

4. Bench Press

Lie flat on a weight bench holding the barbell a bit wider than shoulders-width apart. Lift the barbell from the rack and lower it to just above your chest. Press it back up until your arms are fully extended. Pause, then lower again to begin the next repetition.

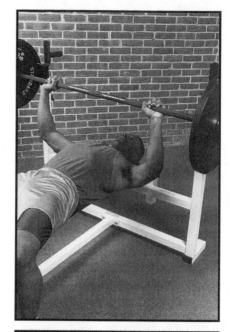

5. Bent-Over Row

Lift barbell off the floor with a narrow grip. Keeping your back parallel to the floor, pull the barbell toward you until it touches your chest. Pause. Then lower.

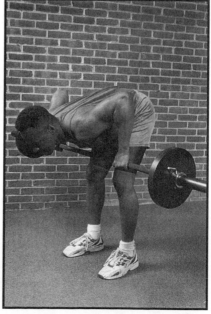

6. Overhead Press

With a shoulders-width grip, lift barbell to your shoulders. Press overhead until arms are fully extended. Pause. Then lower back to shoulders.

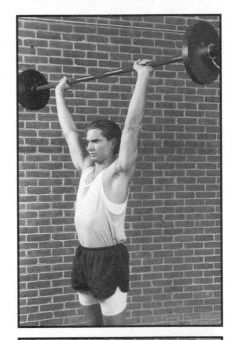

7. Biceps Curl

With an underhand grip, raise barbell to your shoulders. Pause. Then lower.

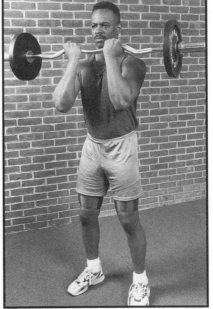

8. Triceps Extension

With a dumbbell in your right hand, and your elbow bent so the dumbbell is behind your head, raise your arm so that it's straight up with the elbow almost locked. Pause, then return to starting position. Repeat set with left arm.

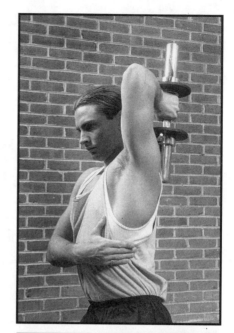

9. Side Bends

With a dumbbell in your right hand, arm hanging straight at your side, place your left hand on your hip and bend at the waist to the right, as far as you can go. Return slowly to original position. Repeat set with the weight in your left hand, bending to the left.

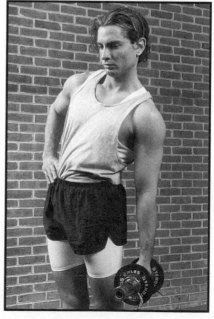

10. Crunches

Lie on your back with your hands behind your head and your knees bent. Keeping your eyes looking straight up at the ceiling, raise—but don't jerk—your head, flattening your stomach muscles. Hold for 2 seconds, then lower.

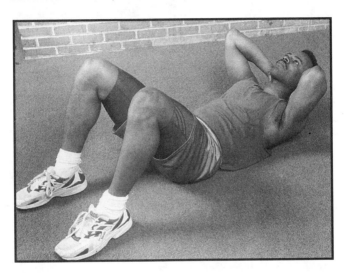

THE LOSE THE LOVE HANDLES CIRCUIT: MACHINE ROUTINE OPTION

Do one set of 10–15 repetitions of each exercise. Then repeat entire circuit 1–2 more times.

To find the weight that's right for you on each lift, first experiment with very light weights, working your way up to a weight that you can lift at least 10 times—but not more than 15 times. That's a good starting weight. Then, when you can easily lift that weight 15 times, add a few pounds.

1. Leg Extension

*Place your ankles
underneath the roller
pads. Place handles on
side grips for stability.
Raise both legs until
knees are straight
(not locked at knee).
Pause. Lower slowly.*

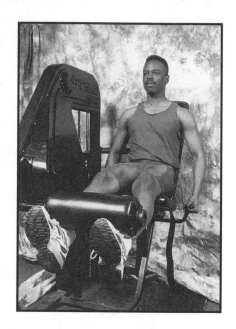

2. Leg Curl

*Lie on your stomach with your knees just over the edge of the
bench and your Achilles tendons hitting the roller pads. Hold
the side grips to prevent your body from sliding. Curl your
legs upward, trying to touch the roller pads to your butt.
Pause. Lower slowly. (If you feel a strain on your lower back,
try one leg at a time.)*

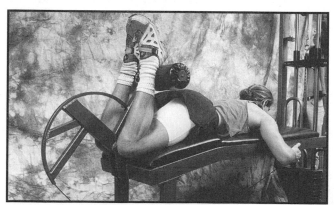

3. Calf Raise

Put belt around your hips and stand up. Grab bar in front of you for stability. Raise up on both feet until you're on your toes. Pause. Lower slowly.

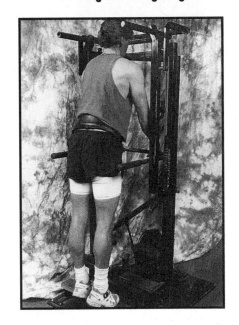

4. Chest Press

Lie flat on the bench, feet flat on the floor and handles in line with your shoulders. With a wide grip, press up until your arms are extended. Pause. Lower slowly.

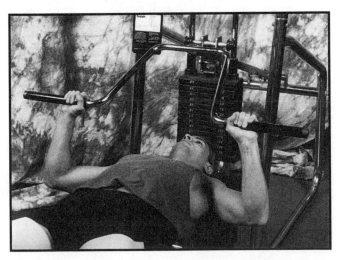

5. Lat Pulldown

Sit with thighs under roller pads for stability. Hold bar behind and slightly above your head with hands about shoulders-width apart. Lower bar behind your head to your shoulders. Pause. Raise slowly.

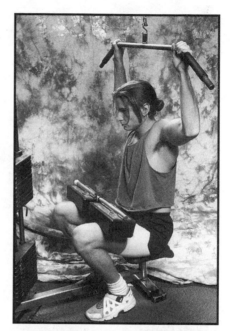

6. Lower Back Extension

Sit in the machine with thighs under roller pads for stability and belt fastened around your waist. Place hands on upper thighs. Push torso backward slowly, as far as you can go. Pause. Return slowly.

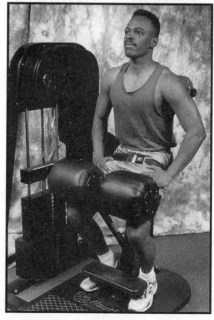

7. Biceps Curl

Sit in the machine with arms outstretched. Grab the handles and bring both arms back toward your shoulders. Pause. Lower slowly.

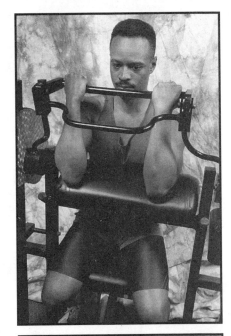

8. Triceps Curl

Sit in the machine with elbows higher than shoulders and arms bent back toward your head. Push on the roller pads with your closed hands to straighten your arms. Pause. Return slowly.

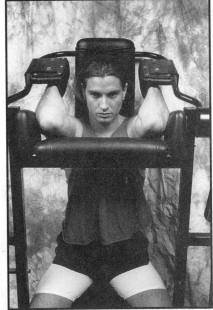

9. Crunches

Sit back in the machine with your hands grasping the handles. Take a deep breath, and exhale while you lean forward at the waist. Be sure you use your stomach muscles to pull the weight, not your arms. Pause. Return slowly.

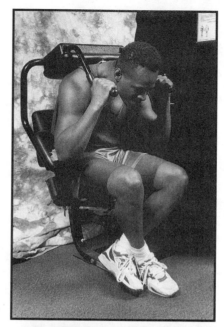

10. Side Bends

Sit upright in the machine with arms behind the roller pads and feet crossed in front of you. Looking straight ahead, twist at the waist until you feel a strain. Pause. Return slowly. Repeat set, twisting to other side.

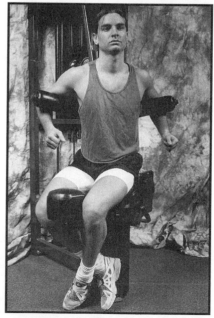

PART 3

EAT TO TRIM

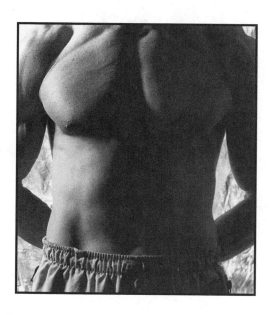

Fuel Your Body in the Battle Against Love Handles!

Dieting . . . slows your metabolism, making it harder for you to burn fat.

Dieting . . . makes you light-headed and weak, making it harder for you to complete the aerobic and weight training parts of the *Losing the Love Handles* program.

Dieting . . . doesn't work. You can't ever *lose* fat cells; you can only shrink them. And every fat cell you shrink by, say, skipping breakfast, is a cell that's eagerly waiting for lunch, waiting for that piece of double-cheese pizza or handful of potato chips to swell it right back up.

That won't happen if you lose your love handles the right way—by using exercise and weight training to make your body a continuously fat-burning machine.

And it won't happen unless you learn to eat sensibly. The *Lose the Love Handles* nutritional program uses food as a weapon in your battle against love handles. This is *not* a diet! You don't have to give up good food! Yes, you can have beer!

Three Squares

Sumo wrestlers have love handles the size of prize watermelons. They *need* them—so that their opponents can't get a good grip around their bodies. Believe it or not, one of the techniques they use to grow those gargantuan handles is skipping breakfast. That drives up hunger and slows the metabolism so that, come lunch, they pack on as much fat as the dozen sushi combo platters they devour.

The point is, skipping any meal or substituting a small snack for a meal is detrimental to your battle against love handles. "You want to avoid hunger—not food," says Nancy Clark, author of *Nancy Clark's Sports Nutrition Guidebook*. The *Lose the Love Handles* nutritional program is based on a dietary proportion of roughly 65 percent carbohydrates, 15 percent protein, and 20 percent fat. You'll be eating the time-honored three square meals a day, plus an optional afternoon snack.

Many fitness programs recommend leaving the table hungry. This program does not take that approach. I repeat: You *will not* go hungry! You'll take your time and eat until your tank is full. You know when you're eating just for pleasure—and not hunger. You'll learn to man the shut-off valve. This will keep your metabolism running at an even burn and will help you avoid hunger pangs, which can lead to overeating, with sumo-sized results.

What to Watch: Calories, Not Necessarily Fat

You could probably lose your love handles on a diet filled with fat (if you ate just a glazed doughnut for breakfast, small fries for lunch, and a slice of pizza for dinner). The point is, dietary fat isn't necessarily your archenemy when you want to lose the handles.

Yes, fatty food is loaded with more calories than non-fatty food. That's why a Big Mac with fries keeps you satiated so long, and vegetables over rice do not. But you can have your fat (which you need to process fat-soluble vitamins and build cell walls) and lose it too. Eating some fat each day keeps you from craving it—then breaking down and dialing Pizza Hut during the *Late Show*. Eating some dietary fat keeps your hunger on an even keel, and lets you concentrate on the real enemy in your battle against love handles: calories.

How to Lose Weight: The Magic of 500

A typical active male, says Clark, burns about 15 calories per pound of body weight each day. That's 2,400 calories burned each day by a 160-pound man, just sitting around. Add to that the calories burned through aerobic exercise and weight lifting, and that daily total can balloon up to 2,700 to 3,400 calories (depending on the length and intensity of the workout).

So to lose weight—to lose those love handles—a 160-pound man simply needs to eat fewer calories than he's burning. A good goal is to eat 500 fewer calories per day than you burn. "If you do that, you'll lose one pound of fat per week," Clark says. In general, for every 3,500 calories you burn and don't replace, your body burns a pound of fat to compensate.

"LIGHTEN" UP

I know. Nothing tastes better after a hard sweaty workout than a cold beer. The most difficult part of losing those handles might be cutting back on that frosted mug reward. But be strong—because alcohol is a major foe in your battle.

Alcohol is *empty* calories, but *preferred* calories. In other words, when alcohol hits your system, your metabolism spends time breaking it down first, shunning other foods that might then get packed on later as fat. You tend to eat extra food when you drink because alcohol stimulates hunger and lowers your inhibitions. Finally, alcohol is a diuretic. It makes you pee and dehydrates you, sending your entire system out of whack.

So when you drink, guys, have a light beer. Or cut a regular beer with ice (as the ice melts, it dilutes your beer, turning it into a de facto light beer and keeping you from being dehydrated in the process). You'll still get that great post-workout reward. But you won't be hindering your efforts to lose the handles.

Skim to Slim

With the *Lose the Love Handles* Nutritional Program you'll be eating three meals a day and even snacking. So where do you cut the extra 500? The answer is: skimming. You won't cut out meals or miss eating what you want. But just by making wise food choices several times a day, you'll easily skim 500 calories from your normal diet. Here's an example of some of those choices and the calories you'll skim:

Skim	Slim
One bowl of Raisin Bran instead of two	220 calories
Water instead of soda, fruit juice, or lemonade	120 to 170 calories
Fruit juice cut with water	60 to 70 calories
Mustard instead of mayonnaise on sandwich	85 calories
Skim milk instead of whole milk	90 calories per cup
No butter or salad dressing	170 calories
Two Oreos instead of four	100 calories
Pretzels instead of potato chips	50 calories per ounce
One tablespoon peanut butter on bagel, not two	100 calories
Vanilla ice cream instead of chocolate Dove Bar	115 calories
Yogurt instead of vanilla ice cream	85 calories

If you're going to eat at restaurants and will be tempted to gorge yourself on good food, the best way to prepare yourself is to snack before going out. Have half a bagel, a banana, or a bag of pretzels. This is especially important if you're eating out after a hard workout. The time it takes you to get ready to go to the restaurant drives hunger way into the danger zone, and you'll be tempted to eat a *lot* of *anything* because "you've earned it."

And that brings up an important point: when to eat following your workout. Try to sit down to a meal as soon as

---

NIGHTTIME HUNGER

You cycled for 20 minutes at tempo pace, did 2 circuits of free weights, had a healthy breakfast, lunch, snack, and dinner. You can feel your love handles melting. But it's 9:30 P.M. *Seinfeld* is over—and you're hungry.

This is what many diet experts refer to as the crisis time. You've just got to suck it up, drink lots of water, and tough it out until morning. Some experts recommend that you eat nothing at all after 8 P.M. (You should drink 8–12 8-ounce glasses of water a day. You'll need the fluids to replace what you lost to sweat. Water also helps you feel less hungry—it fills up the stomach.)

The *Lose the Love Handles* nutritional program is not nearly so monastic. "You can eat," says Nancy Clark. "As long as you don't overeat." A good nighttime snack is something light, preferably high in carbohydrates (carbohydrates contain tryptophan, an amino acid that helps bring on sleep). Half a bagel is good; so is a bowl of cereal (as long as it's not sugarcoated). Cold pasta left over from dinner can quell your hunger, or a piece of fruit.

Chips, ice cream, and cookies are not wise choices at this time, but let's hope you won't be craving fatty foods late at night because you'll have eaten some fat during the day. If you do have a weakness for these foods, the secret is not to buy them: Don't have them in the house. If late-night pizza is your Achilles' heel, tear out the Yellow Pages for pizza delivery from your phone book. Let 'er *ripppp!*

possible, for two reasons: 1) your metabolism will be at a high point and so you'll naturally burn more of your meal off; and 2) your hunger pangs will be lowest. You will actually be hungrier one hour after your workout than 20 minutes after—so you will eat less the sooner you eat.

PART 4

YOUR DAILY LOG

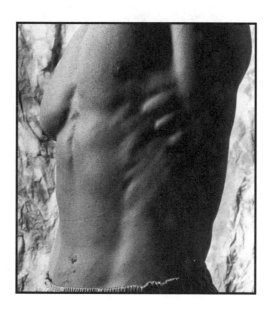

THE ONE-MONTH COUNTDOWN

Your *Lose the Love Handles* daily log is invaluable. It will help you keep track of your progress, and it lets you record the work you're doing toward an arrow-straight waist. It also serves as a motivational tool. You'll look forward to filling in a workout each day because it gives you a sense of pride and accomplishment. Blank spaces in your log don't look so hot.

The log is divided into two sections: *Sweat* and *Fuel*. The *Sweat* section contains the exercise goal for that day as found in Part 1. Then there's a space for you to fill in the actual workout you completed that day. Try, of course, to make the two match as closely as possible. Finally, fill in the number of weight circuits you completed that day (if it's a day you were scheduled to lift weights). The *Fuel* section shows you the food you'll be eating that day to help power you through your workouts.

Work hard. And don't forget to have fun—try new ways to work up a sweat. You're on your way to losing the handles in 30 days!

DAY 1 / MONDAY

SWEAT

Exercise Goal: 20-minute tempo ride (85 percent)

Exercise Actual: _____

Weight Circuits: _____

FUEL

Breakfast: Cereal with skim milk, banana, 4-ounce glass of fruit juice cut with 4 ounces of water.

Lunch: Turkey with mustard and one slice Swiss cheese on whole-wheat bread, pretzels, water.

Snack: Poppy seed bagel, plain.

Dinner: Spaghetti with kidney beans, tomato sauce, steamed broccoli, glass of skim milk, two Oreos.

DAY 2/TUESDAY

SWEAT

Exercise Goal: 20 minutes easy

Exercise Actual: _____

FUEL

Breakfast: Pancakes with applesauce, 4-ounce glass of fruit juice cut with 4 ounces of water.

Lunch: Slice of French bread pizza, fruit juice cut with water.

Snack: No snack because of fatty lunch.

Dinner: Chicken breast on rice, green beans, glass of skim milk.

DAY 3/**WEDNESDAY**

SWEAT

Exercise Goal: 25 minutes easy

Exercise Actual: _____

FUEL

Breakfast: Cereal with skim milk, banana, water.

Lunch: Cup of yogurt, bagel, fruit juice cut with water.

Snack: Apple.

Dinner: Baked fish with lemon, baked potato, salad, skim milk, two cookies.

DAY 4/**THURSDAY**

SWEAT

Exercise Goal: Run 4 × 60 seconds at 90–95 percent

Exercise Actual: _____

Weight Circuits: _____

FUEL

Breakfast: Bagel with dab of peanut butter, bowl of cereal, glass of fruit juice cut with water.

Lunch: Tuna fish sandwich, pretzels, water.

Snack: Banana.

Dinner: Red beans and rice, salad, glass of skim milk, cup of yogurt.

DAY 5/FRIDAY

SWEAT

Exercise Goal: 30 minutes easy

Exercise Actual: _____

FUEL

Breakfast: Oatmeal with banana, fruit juice cut with water.

Lunch: Turkey with mustard and one slice Swiss cheese on whole-wheat bread, pretzels, water.

Snack: Plain bagel.

Dinner: Stir-fried beef and broccoli over rice, glass of skim milk, brownie.

DAY 6/**SATURDAY**

SWEAT

Exercise Goal: Cycle 50 minutes at 75 percent effort

Exercise Actual: _____

FUEL

Breakfast: Two frozen waffles, syrup, banana, fruit juice cut with water.

Lunch: Chef's salad with light dressing, water.

Snack: Cup of yogurt.

Dinner: Lasagne, two slices whole-grain bread, unbuttered, glass of skim milk, two cookies.

DAY 7/SUNDAY

SWEAT

None. Take a nap.

FUEL

Breakfast: Cereal, banana, glass of water.

Lunch: Lean roast beef sandwich, no cheese, pretzels, fruit juice cut with water.

Snack: Bagel.

Dinner: Spaghetti with kidney beans, tomato sauce, steamed broccoli, glass of skim milk, two Oreos.

DAY 8/MONDAY

SWEAT

Exercise Goal: Stairclimb 23 minutes at 85 percent effort

Exercise Actual: ⎯⎯⎯⎯⎯⎯⎯⎯⎯

Weight Circuits: ⎯⎯⎯⎯⎯⎯⎯⎯

FUEL

Breakfast: Pancakes with applesauce, fruit juice cut with water.

Lunch: Bowl of soup, bagel, water.

Snack: Pretzels.

Dinner: Chicken breast on rice, green beans, glass of skim milk.

DAY 9/TUESDAY

SWEAT

Exercise Goal: 20 minutes easy

Exercise Actual: _____

FUEL

Breakfast: Toasted bagel with peanut butter, grapefruit, water.

Lunch: Turkey with mustard and one slice Swiss cheese on whole-wheat bread, pretzels, water.

Snack: Banana.

Dinner: Baked fish with lemon, baked potato, salad, skim milk.

DAY 1 0/**WEDNESDAY**

SWEAT

Exercise Goal: 25 minutes easy

Exercise Actual: _____

FUEL

Breakfast: Egg Beaters sandwich (two Egg Beaters scrambled inside a bagel or two pieces of bread), banana, fruit juice cut with water.

Lunch: Tuna fish sandwich, carrot stick, fruit juice cut with water.

Snack: Apple.

Dinner: Red beans and rice, salad, glass of skim milk, cup of yogurt.

DAY 11/**THURSDAY**

SWEAT

Exercise Goal: Run 5 × 60 seconds at 95 percent effort

Exercise Actual: _____

Weight Circuits: _____

FUEL

Breakfast: Frozen waffles, syrup, grapefruit, water.

Lunch: Chef's salad with light dressing, fruit juice cut with water.

Snack: Cup of yogurt.

Dinner: Lasagne, two slices of bread, salad, skim milk, two cookies.

DAY 12/FRIDAY

SWEAT

Exercise Goal: 20 minutes easy

Exercise Actual: _____

FUEL

Breakfast: Cereal, banana, fruit juice cut with water.

Lunch: Lean roast beef sandwich, pretzels, water.

Snack: Bagel.

Dinner: Stir-fried beef and broccoli over rice, salad, skim milk, brownie.

DAY 13/SATURDAY

SWEAT

Exercise Goal: Cycle 60 minutes at 75 percent effort

Exercise Actual: _____

FUEL

Breakfast: Pancakes with applesauce, fruit juice cut with water.

Lunch: One slice French bread pizza, water.

Snack: Pretzels.

Dinner: Chicken breast on rice, green beans, skim milk.

DAY 14/SUNDAY

SWEAT

None.

FUEL

Breakfast: Toasted bagel with peanut butter, grapefruit, water.

Lunch: Turkey with mustard and one slice Swiss cheese on whole-wheat bread, pretzels, fruit juice cut with water.

Snack: Banana.

Dinner: Spaghetti with kidney beans, tomato sauce, steamed broccoli, skim milk, two Oreos.

DAY 1 5/MONDAY

SWEAT

Exercise Goal: Run 27 minutes at 85 percent

Exercise Actual: _____

Weight Circuits: _____

FUEL

Breakfast: Egg Beaters sandwich, banana, fruit juice cut with water.

Lunch: Soup, bagel, water.

Snack: Apple.

Dinner: Baked fish with lemon, baked potato, salad, skim milk.

DAY 16/**TUESDAY**

SWEAT

Exercise Goal: 25 minutes easy

Exercise Actual: _____

FUEL

Breakfast: Smoothie (banana and strawberries blended with orange juice), bagel, water.

Lunch: Tuna fish sandwich, pretzels, fruit juice cut with water.

Snack: Yogurt.

Dinner: Red beans and rice, salad, skim milk, yogurt.

DAY 17/WEDNESDAY

SWEAT

Exercise Goal: 20 minutes easy

Exercise Actual: _____

FUEL

Breakfast: Oatmeal with banana, fruit juice cut with water.

Lunch: Lean roast beef sandwich with slice of Swiss cheese, carrot stick, water.

Snack: Bagel.

Dinner: Macaroni and cheese and mixed vegetables, skim milk, brownie.

DAY 18/**THURSDAY**

SWEAT

Exercise Goal: Run 6 × 60 seconds at 95 percent effort

Exercise Actual: _____

Weight Circuits: _____

FUEL

Breakfast: Frozen waffles, syrup, grapefruit, water.

Lunch: Chef's salad, fruit juice cut with water.

Snack: Pretzels.

Dinner: Lasagne, two slices of bread, glass of skim milk, two cookies.

DAY 19/**FRIDAY**

SWEAT

Exercise Goal: 20 minutes easy

Exercise Actual: _____

FUEL

Breakfast: Cereal, banana, fruit juice cut with water.

Lunch: Soup, bagel, water.

Snack: Banana.

Dinner: Chicken breast on rice, green beans, skim milk.

DAY 2O/SATURDAY

SWEAT

Exercise Goal: Stairclimb 60 minutes at 75 percent effort

Exercise Actual: _____

FUEL

Breakfast: Pancakes with applesauce, fruit juice cut with water.

Lunch: Turkey with mustard and one slice Swiss cheese on whole-wheat bread, pretzels, fruit juice cut with water.

Snack: Apple.

Dinner: Make-your-own veggie pizza (easy on the cheese), skim milk, two Oreos.

DAY 21/SUNDAY

SWEAT

None.

FUEL

Breakfast: Toasted bagel with peanut butter, grapefruit, water.

Lunch: Tuna fish sandwich, pretzels, fruit juice cut with water.

Snack: Yogurt.

Dinner: Baked fish with lemon, baked potato, salad, skim milk, two cookies.

DAY 22/MONDAY

SWEAT

Exercise Goal: Cycle 30 minutes at 85 percent effort

Exercise Actual: _____

Weight Circuits: _____

FUEL

Breakfast: Egg Beaters sandwich, banana, fruit juice cut with water.

Lunch: Lean roast beef sandwich with Swiss cheese, carrots and celery, water.

Snack: Bagel.

Dinner: Spaghetti and meat sauce, salad, French bread (easy on the butter), skim milk.

DAY 23/**TUESDAY**

SWEAT

Exercise Goal: 20 minutes easy

Exercise Actual: _____

FUEL

Breakfast: Smoothie, bagel, water.

Lunch: Soup, bagel, fruit juice cut with water.

Snack: Pretzels.

Dinner: Ground-turkey burger with all the fixin's, baked potato, skim milk, two cookies.

DAY 24/**WEDNESDAY**

SWEAT

Exercise Goal: 20 minutes easy

Exercise Actual: _____

FUEL

Breakfast: Oatmeal with banana, fruit juice cut with water.

Lunch: Chef's salad with light dressing, fruit juice cut with water.

Snack: Banana.

Dinner: Stir-fried beef and broccoli over rice, salad, skim milk.

DAY 25/THURSDAY

SWEAT

Exercise Goal: 7 × 60 seconds at 95 percent effort

Exercise Actual: _____

Weight Circuits: _____

FUEL

Breakfast: Cereal, grapefruit, water.

Lunch: Turkey sandwich with one slice Swiss cheese, pretzels, fruit juice cut with water.

Snack: Apple.

Dinner: Spaghetti with kidney beans, tomato sauce, steamed broccoli, skim milk, two Oreos.

DAY 26/**F**RIDAY

SWEAT

Exercise Goal: 20 minutes easy

Exercise Actual: _____

FUEL

Breakfast: Toasted bagel with peanut butter, banana, water.

Lunch: Tuna fish sandwich, pretzels, fruit juice cut with water.

Snack: Yogurt.

Dinner: Grilled chicken breast sandwich (easy on the mayo), oven-baked French fries, skim milk, two cookies.

DAY 27/SATURDAY

SWEAT

Exercise Goal: Cycle 60 minutes at 75 percent effort

Exercise Actual: _____

FUEL

Breakfast: Pancakes with applesauce, fruit juice cut with water.

Lunch: Lean roast beef sandwich, pretzels, water.

Snack: Bagel.

Dinner: Baked fish with lemon, baked potato, salad, skim milk, two cookies.

DAY 28/SUNDAY

SWEAT

None.

FUEL

Breakfast: Frozen waffles, syrup, grapefruit, water.

Lunch: Soup, bagel, fruit juice cut with water.

Snack: Pretzels.

Dinner: Red beans and rice, salad, milk, yogurt.

DAY 29/MONDAY

SWEAT

Exercise Goal: Stairclimb 30 minutes at 85 percent effort

Exercise Actual: _____

Weight Circuits: _____

FUEL

Breakfast: Egg Beaters sandwich, banana, fruit juice cut with water.

Lunch: Large slice of cheese pizza, fruit juice.

Snack: Banana.

Dinner: Lasagne, two slices of bread, milk, two cookies.

DAY 30/**TUESDAY**

SWEAT

Exercise Goal: 20 minutes easy

Exercise Actual: _____

FUEL

Breakfast: Cereal, banana, fruit juice cut with water.

Lunch: Turkey sandwich with one slice Swiss cheese, pretzels, fruit juice cut with water.

Snack: Apple.

Dinner: Stir-fried beef and broccoli over rice, salad, skim milk.

NOTES

NOTES

ABOUT THE AUTHOR

Dave Kuehls, a senior writer at *Runner's World* magazine, writes frequently for such publications as *GQ, Sports Illustrated, Men's Health,* and *Outside.* Co-author of *The Runner's Book of Training Secrets,* he is an avid follower of the *Lose the Love Handles* program and has an arrow-straight waist. He lives in Akron, Ohio.